LITTLE BOOK OF PELVIC
FLOOR POWER

ANNE SHIRLEY HOSELTON

LITTLE BOOK OF PELVIC FLOOR POWER

Fort Diaz Press

TABLE OF CONTENTS

PELVIC FLOOR

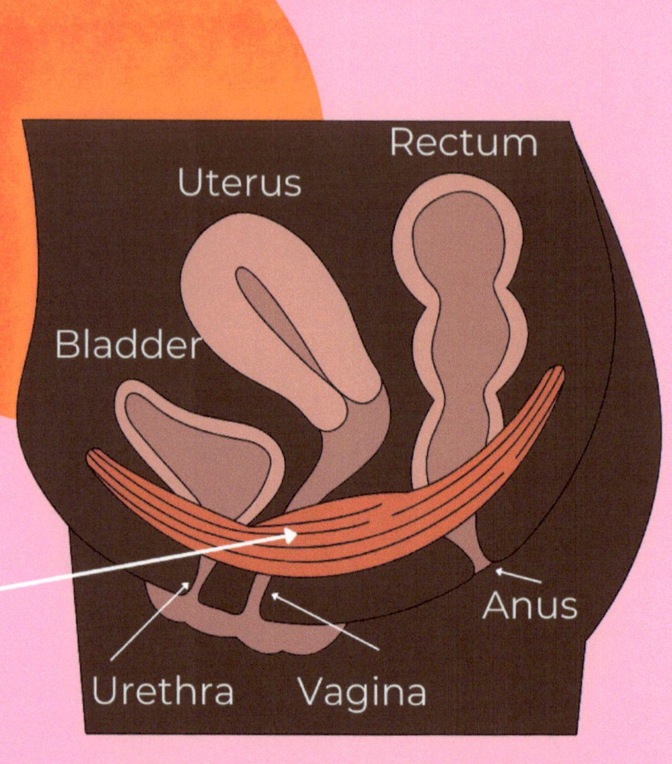

This diagram is a cross-sectional view of the female pelvis. From front to back, there is the urethra & bladder, vagina & uterus, and anus & rectum. The pelvic floor is the group of muscles at the interface between the pelvic organs and their respective outlets. As such, the pelvic floor plays an important role in urinary continence, sexual function, and fecal continence.

PELVIC FLOOR DYSFUNCTION

Pelvic Floor Dysfunction is a broad term for any problems that may arise due to abnormal function of the pelvic floor. Conditions may include:

Urinary incontinence

Cystocele (bulging of bladder into vagina)

Dyspareunia (pain with sex)

Uterine prolapse

Vaginal prolapse

Rectocele (bulging of rectum into vagina)

Constipation

Fecal incontinence

Rectal prolapse

Many conditions of pelvic floor dysfunction can be improved with self-paced pelvic floor exercises or focused pelvic floor physical therapy. However, some conditions may require surgical intervention to improve symptoms. Talk with your doctor if you have any questions about management of pelvic floor dysfunction.

PREGNANCY & THE PELVIC FLOOR

While pelvic floor dysfunction can affect anyone, pregnancy and childbirth are significant risk factors.

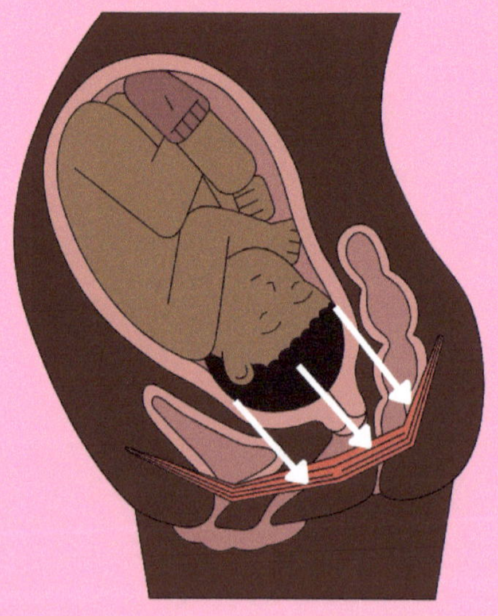

Throughout pregnancy, the growing uterus puts pressure on the pelvic floor muscles. During vaginal delivery, the muscles are further stretched to accommodate passage of the baby through the birth canal. The result is that pelvic floor muscles may be weakened, increasing the likelihood of pelvic floor dysfunction.

PELVIC FLOOR EXERCISE

The following pages contain a self-paced program of movements that help to target the pelvic floor. To start...

WHAT IS A KEGEL?

You may have heard of Kegels. A Kegel (pronounced "kay-gl") is a voluntary contraction of the muscles of the pelvic floor. A regular practice of Kegels can help to strengthen the pelvic floor and prevent or improve symptoms of pelvic floor dysfunction.

How to do an effective Kegel

Locate your pelvic floor muscles. The best way to do this is to stop urinating mid-stream. The muscles that contract to stop your stream of urine are your pelvic floor muscles, and the action of squeezing off the urine stream is very similar to a Kegel!

Next, practice this contraction. You can do this almost anywhere. Get comfortable and focus on squeezing your pelvic muscles. You can picture trying to squeeze a marble in your vagina. It may help to insert a finger in the vagina to feel the contraction. Make sure that the contraction is coming from your pelvic floor, and not from your buttocks or abdominal muscles.

HOW TO USE

Mix and match exercises from each category to design your own workout

Repeat each exercise for the specified number of repetitions

Do 3-5 days/week for improved pelvic floor strength!

IT WILL LOOK LIKE THIS:

1 Kegel Warm-up

2 Choose 1 Tuck

3 Choose 1 Squat

4 Choose 1 Supine

5 Choose 1 Bridge

6 Choose 1 Hands & Knees

7 Choose 1 Challenge

8 Kegel Finisher

9 Cool-down

START HERE:

(Refer to page 4 for a full
description of how to do a Kegel))

Kegel Warm-Up

Get in a comfortable position.
You can be seated in a chair or
lying comfortably on your back.

Focus on the small muscles of
your pelvic floor.

Contract your pelvic floor
muscles into the tightest
possible Kegel.

Hold for 5 sec
Relax for 5 sec
Hold for 5 sec
Relax for 5 sec
Hold for 10 sec
} Repeat 3x

A few notes on Kegels:

Your glute and abdominal muscles should not
be contracting when you do a Kegel. Focus on
relaxing those muscles so that you can isolate
the pelvic floor muscles.

Kegels are exercise! Don't be surprised if you
feel your muscles fatiguing or if you notice
some soreness the next day. As you continue
your practice, the muscles will get stronger.

CHOOSE 1 TUCK

Option 1: Lying Tuck

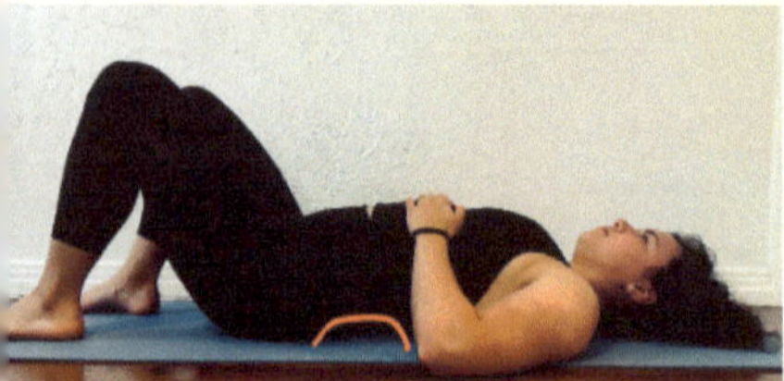

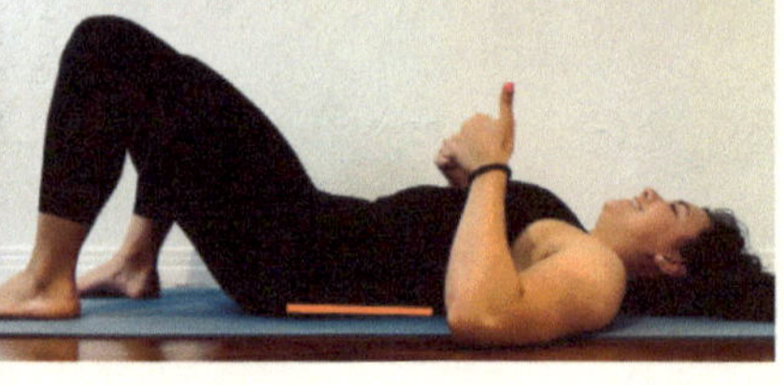

Start laying on your back with your feet planted on the ground. For most women, this position has a natural anterior pelvic tilt, which means that there will be a space between your low back and the floor. The movement is a pelvic tilt, which engages the lower abdominal muscles and the pelvic floor. Think about tilting your pelvis posteriorly until your low back is fully on the ground, and there is no space between your low back and the ground. This is the same movement you would do if you were sitting up straight in a chair and then started to slide your bottom off the seat of the chair. Make sure the motion is coming from your lower abdominal muscles, and not your glutes or thighs!

Hold tuck for 5 sec, then relax. Repeat 10x

Option 2: Standing Tuck

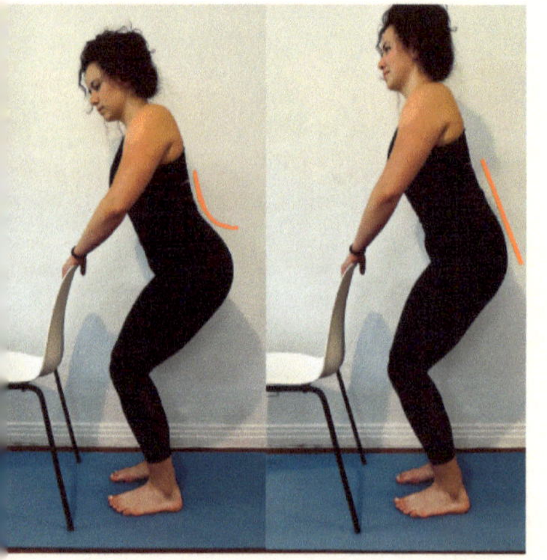

Option 3: Plié Tuck

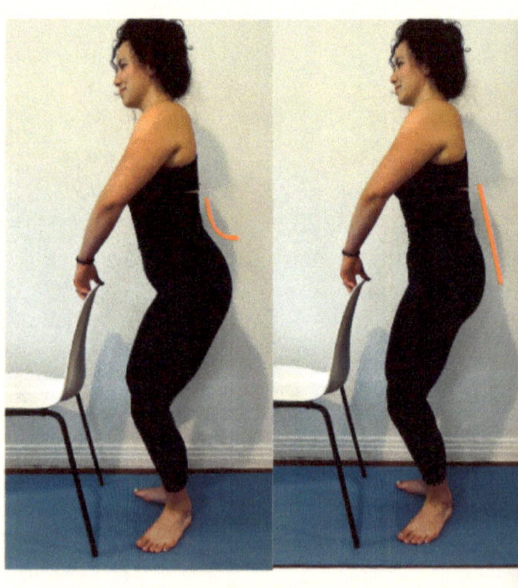

Stand holding a chair, couch, or counter for stability. Plant your feet straight under you, hip-distance apart. Maintain a slight bend at the knees and at the hips. Arch your back to push your tailbone away from you. (This is the same motion as a squat or twerk) From there, roll your hips up and under into a tucked position.

Hold tuck for 5 sec, then relax. Repeat 10x

Very similar to standing tucks. Instead of keeping your feet hip-distance apart, have your heels together and your toes apart. In ballet, this is referred to as first position. Start with your back arched. From there, engage the lower abdominal muscles to tightly tuck the pelvis.

Hold tuck for 5 sec, then relax. Repeat 10x

CHOOSE 1 SQUAT

Option 1: Sit-to-Stand

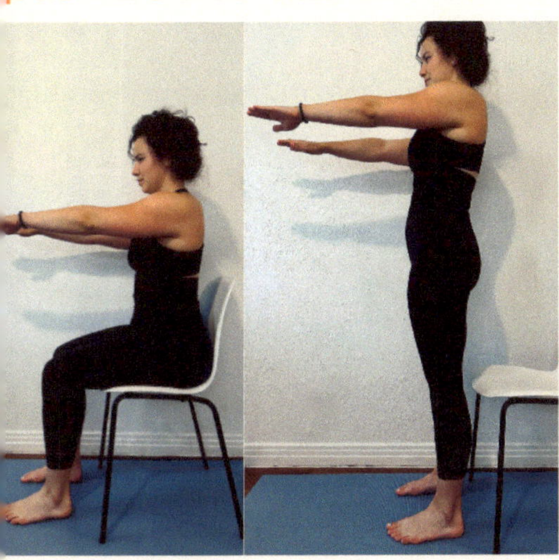

You will need a chair, couch, or bench. Start in seated position. Without using your arms or momentum, slowly lift yourself to standing. Slowly lower yourself back to seated position. Resist gravity to prevent yourself from just falling back into the seat. Move slowly and with control. Think about maintaining tight abdominal muscles throughout the entire movement.

Repeat 10x

Option 2: Squat Pulse

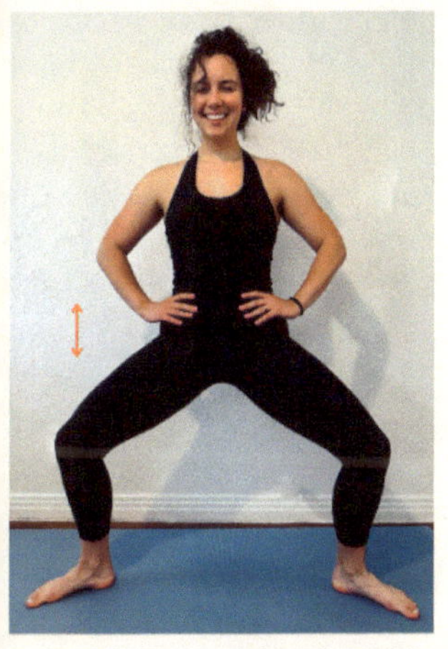

...nd with legs wider than hip ...tance. Heels towards the center and ...es pointing out. Lower into a squat ...u can start with a shallow squat and ...rk towards deepening the squat as ...u progress.) While in a squatting ...sition, do 10 slow pulses up and ...wn. The pulses are small movements ... and down, and not a full squat. After ...ulses, straighten legs to stand. ...intain your **tucked** pelvis!

squat pulses. Repeat 5x

Option 3: Lunge with Rotation

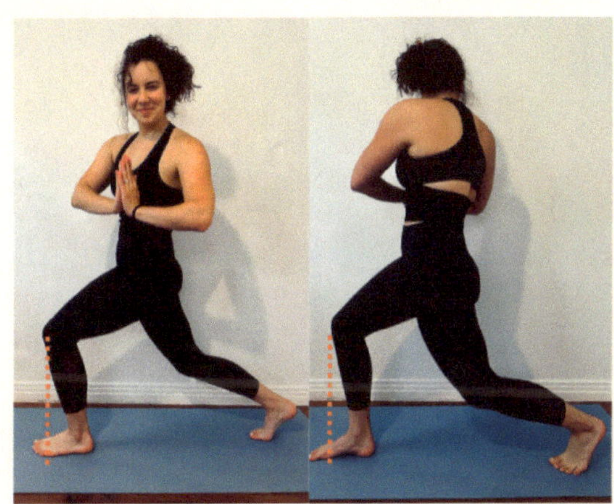

Start in standing position with feet hip-distance apart. Step one foot back into a lunge. Make sure that the front knee does not come past your front toes. With your hands in prayer position, slowly rotate your upper body over the front knee and then back to starting position. Return legs to standing position. Switch legs and rotate the upper body the opposite direction. Move slowly and with control. Keep those hips **tucked**!

Repeat 5x on each side

CHOOSE 1 SUPINE

Option 1: Table Top (with towel)

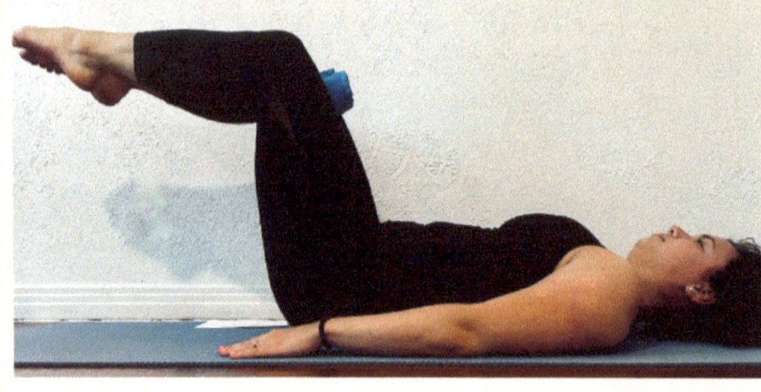

You will need a rolled towel (or other compressible item). Start in table top position, with your back **flat** on the ground. (keep it tucked!) Place the towel between your knees. Squeeze the knees and thighs together to compress the towel.

Squeeze 5 sec. Repeat 10x

Option 2: Toe Tap

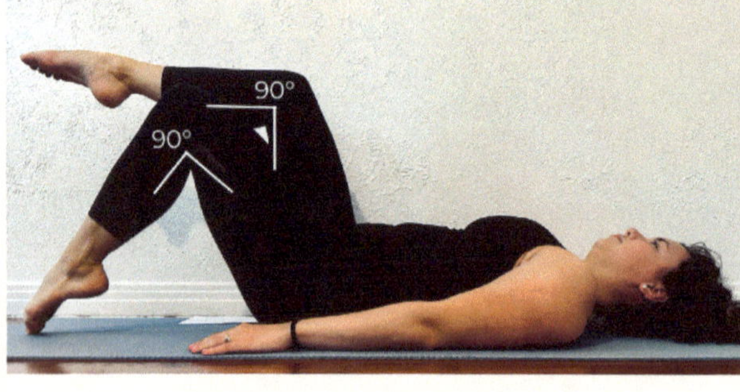

Start lying on your back with your lower abdomen engaged (no space under low back). Lift your legs into table-top positio with the directly over the hips and at a 90° angle. Keep the knee locked in the 90° angle. **Slowly** lower one thigh-leg uni down until the toe touches the ground, then lift back to startir position. Do not let the low bac lift off from the ground.

Repeat 10x on each side

Option 3: Dead Bugs

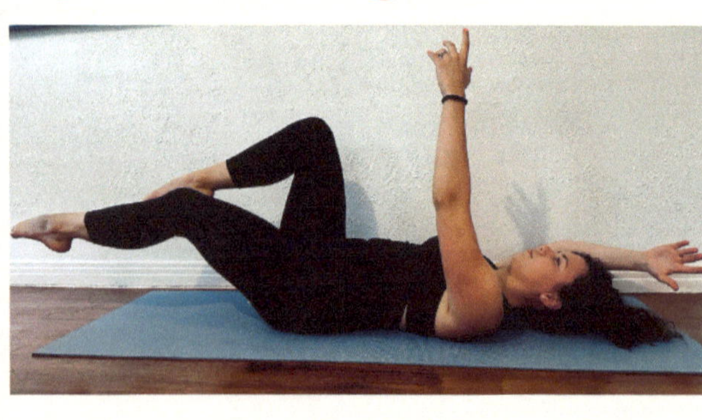

Start in table-top position, with feet off the floor and knees bent at 90°. Hold your arms in front of you like a zombie. While one leg extends out long, the opposite arm is lowered above the head. Both limbs then return to the starting position. Keep that low back on the ground the **entire** time. You will feel the burn.

Repeat 10x on each side

CHOOSE 1 BRIDGE

Option 1: Bridge

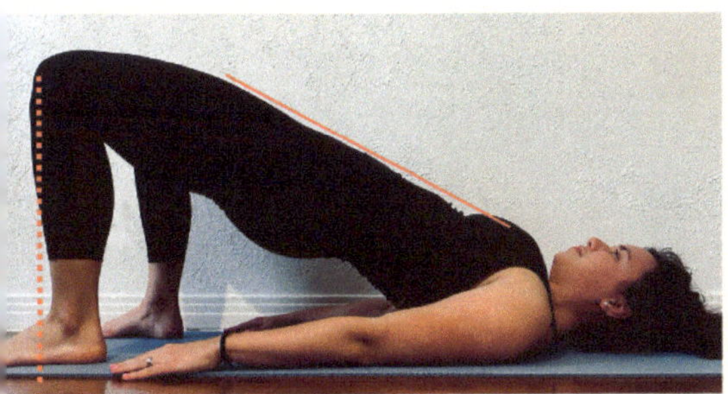

Lie on your back with your feet planted on the ground. Squeeze your glutes to raise your bottom off the ground into a high bridge. Try to make a straight line from your chest to your knees. Keep your knees behind your toes.

Hold bridge for 5 sec. Relax. Repeat 10x

Option 2: Bridge with Adduction and Abduction

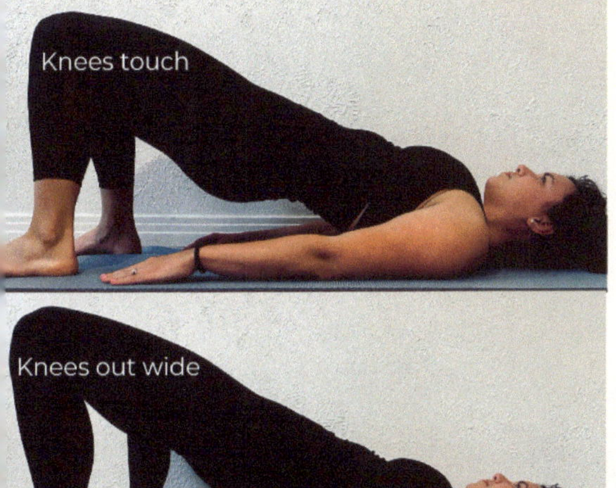

Hold bridge position as above. You can lift onto your tippy-toes for a challenge or stay on flat feet. Once in high bridge, adduct (pull together) your knees until they touch. Then abduct (pull apart) your knees slightly wider than starting position. Maintain high hips through both movements. Return to neutral bridge position and lower down.

Lift into high bridge, touch knees together, then pull them wide. Lower down. Repeat 10x

Option 3: Bridge March

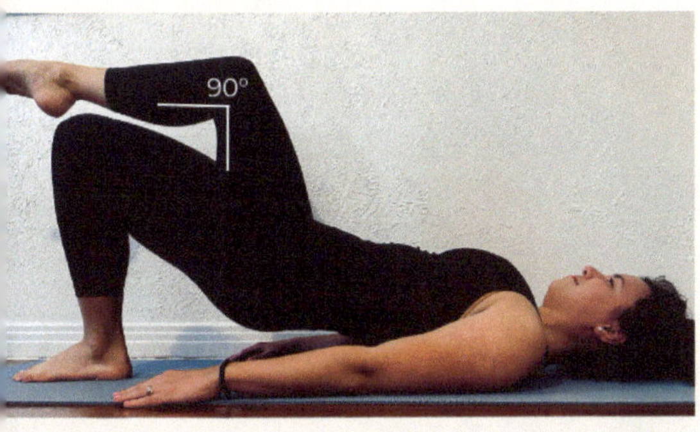

Lift into bridge position. Slowly lift one foot off the ground until it reaches table top position at 90°. Slowly lower leg down. Repeat with opposite leg. Maintain high hips throughout the movement.

Lift into high bridge, lift right leg, then lift left leg. Lower down. Repeat 10x

CHOOSE 1 HANDS & KNEES

Option 1: Cat-Cow

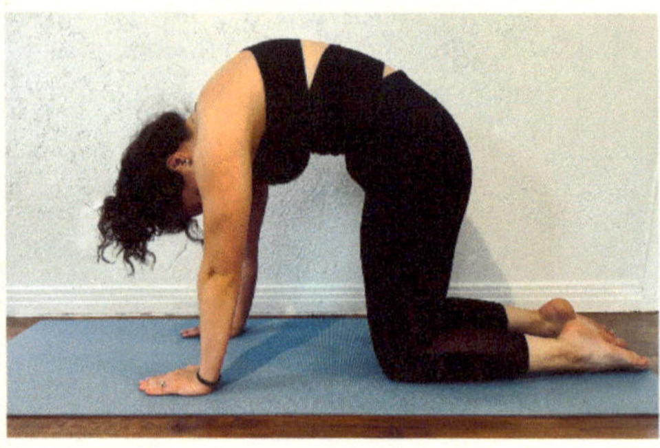 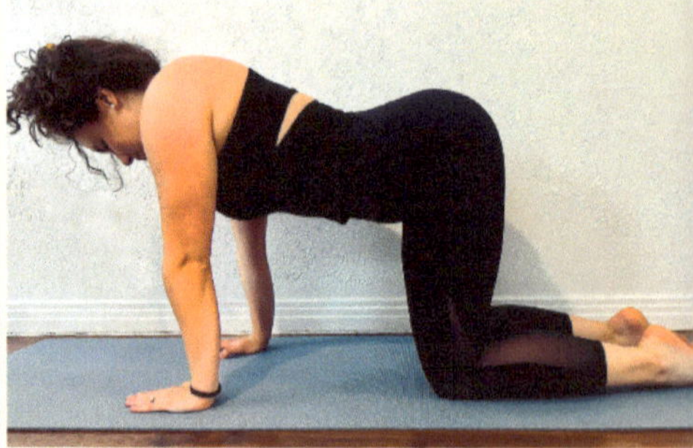

Start on your hands and knees. First, flex your back upwards into your best impression of a scared cat. Let the head dangle down in line with the spine.

Next, arch your back for your best impression of a sway-backed cow. You can arch your neck up so that you are looking at the ceiling. Take your time and enjoy the stretches.

Repeat sequence 10x slowly

Option 2: Bird-Dogs

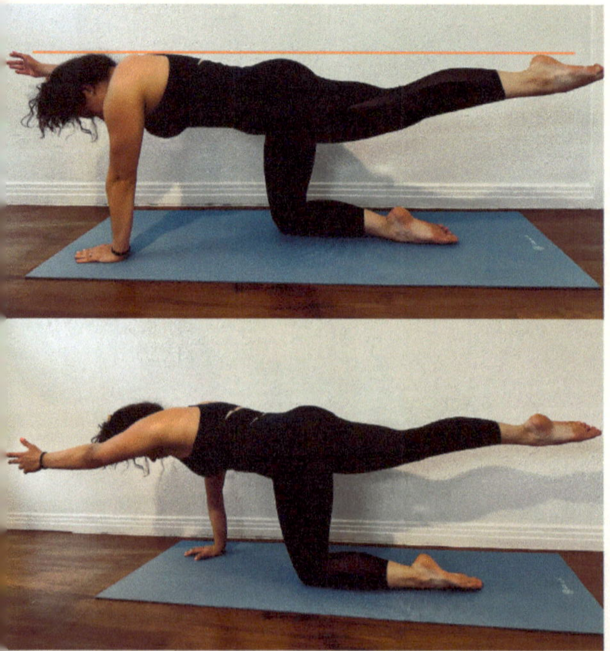

Start on your hands and knees. Extend one leg up in line with t body. Slowly extend the opposi arm out in front. Try to maintair straight line from the tip if your fingertips to the tip of your toes Focus on keeping your hips tucked. Return to starting position on your hands and knees. Repeat the motion with the opposite leg and arm.

Repeat 10x on each side

CHOOSE 1 CHALLENGE

Option 1: Clam

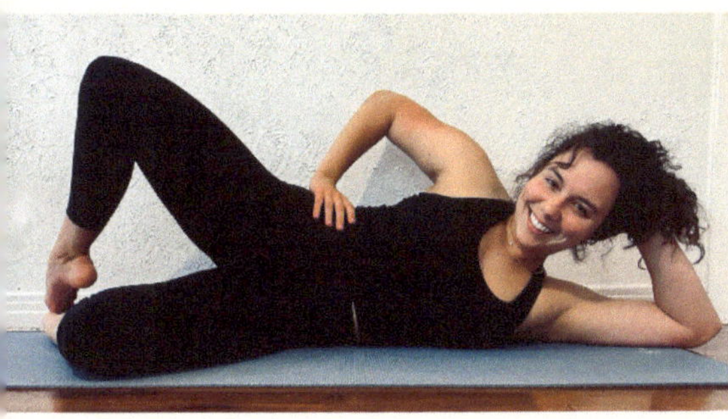

Start lying on your side. You can prop your head up with your arm or lay your head flat. Pull your knees up in a 90° angle in front of you. While keeping your toes touching, slowly open the top leg up like a "clam shell." Hold the clam position for 3 seconds, then return the leg on top of the other leg.

Hold for 5 sec. Repeat 10x each side

Option 2: Heel Slide

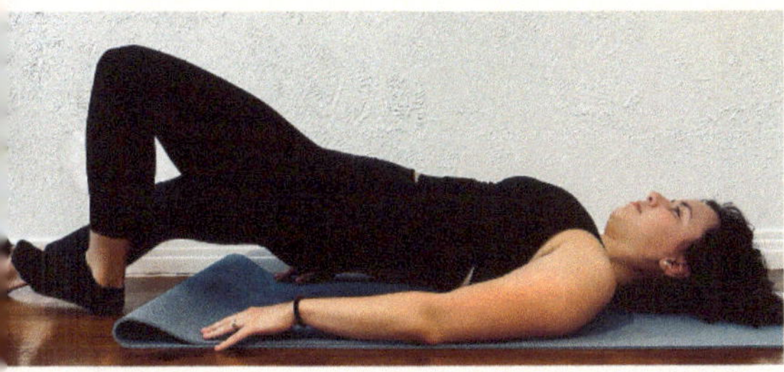

You may need socks on a smooth surface. Lift into a high bridge position. Slowly slide one of your heels away from you until the leg is straightened. Then slowly slide the heel back to starting position. Try to maintain the high bridge position throughout the movement.

Repeat 5x each side

Option 3: Prone Diamond

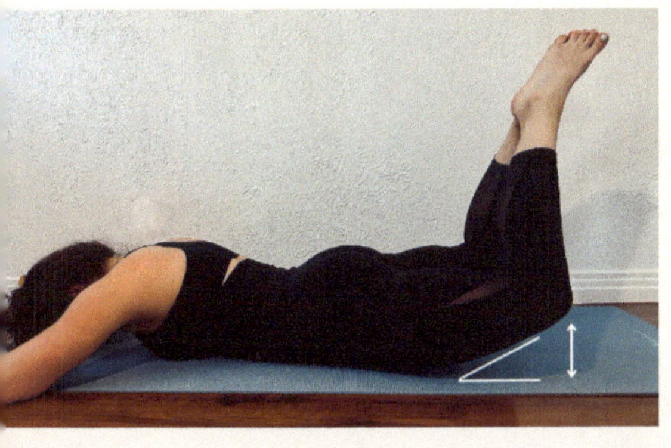

Start lying face-down with your head resting on your hands. Spread your knees apart and touch the soles of your feet together to make a diamond (or froggy leg) position. Engage the low back and glute muscles to lift your thighs off the floor while maintaining the diamond shape with your feet and legs.

Hold for 5 sec. Repeat x10

KEGEL FINISHER

It's time for those kegels again!

Get in a comfortable position. You can be seated in a chair or lying comfortable on your back.

Focus on the small muscles of your pelvic floor.

Contract your pelvic floor muscles into the tightest possible Kegel.

Hold for 5 sec
Relax for 5 sec
Hold for 5 sec
Relax for 5 sec
Hold for 10 sec

} Repeat 3x

COOL-DOWN

YOU DESERVE THIS ONE!

Child's Pose

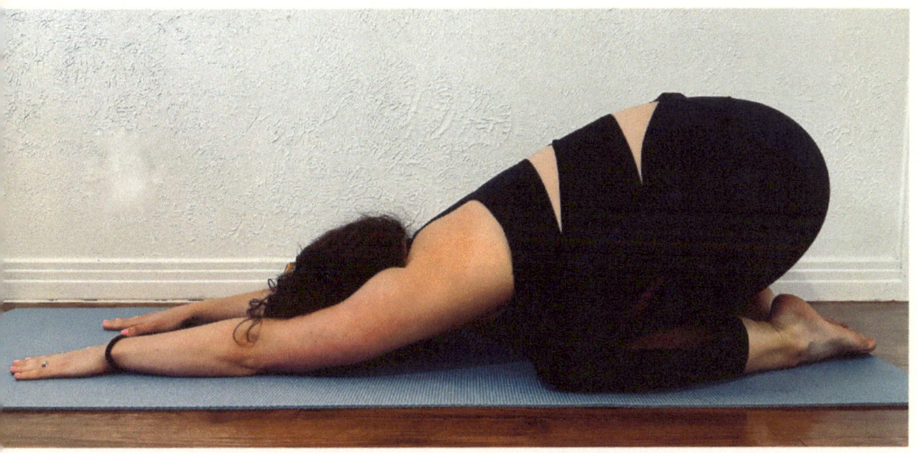

Start on your hands and knees. Adjust your legs so that your feet touch while your knees remain apart. Sink back so that you are resting your weight on your legs, with your arms outstretched. Take slow, deep breaths in this position. You may deepen the stretch by slowly shifting your knees farther apart and letting your hips sink closer to the ground. You can also move your arms slowly to each side for a good side stretch.

Hold for at least 5 slow and controlled breaths

NOTES:

Track your progress here. How do you feel? What went well? What didn't go well? Which movements were most challenging? What are your goals moving forward?

____

____

____

____

____

____

____

____

____

____

____

____

____

____

NOTES:

NOTES:

NOTES: